TLP Starting Line
Life Planning Manual

TERRY MILLER

Requests for information or orders contact:
Miller Tribe Publishing, c/o The Sound 651 W. Sunflower Ave., Santa Ana, CA 92707 or 714.546.8911

www.TotalLifePursuit.org

First edition: April 2020

ISBN-13: 978-0-9912579-2-8

There are many people to thank for their help with this manual, but first and foremost I have to give thanks to God. Father, you have stirred me, inspired me, encouraged me, equipped me and put me in the right place at the right time to learn, grow and have the time to produce this manual. I can't thank you enough.

There also have been many people who have contributed to the making of this manual, one way or another. First a big shout out to Ashley, my editor and really co-writer at times. You have been the biggest cheerleader at my table and I appreciate you so much. Without you this would still be a rough draft in a computer folder. Kimberly, who was my district supervisor for years, helped me to go after the types of conceptions that are in this manual. She opened my eyes to a new way of planning, and not only taught me many things that are within these pages, but she stirred me to learn more. I must have bought ten books after the course that she gave us on planning. Thank you Pastor Brian for giving me the opportunity to work this material out with the people we pastor as well as believe in the entire concept and ministry of Total Life Pursuit. The freedom to write and produce content has been a Godsend.

There are so many people who have poured into me over the years. I have had great mentors like Dave Poc, and Kimberly, I have been to conferences and seminars, I have read articles and books, and there have been people, as I was teaching the concepts in this manual, who gave me helpful corrections. Zoe, my daughter, who is my assistant is invaluable to me. I would have never had the time or focus to finish this manual without you. I owe my entire family gratitude for forcing me to be a planner. With eight children, if you don't have a plan, you have chaos. Perhaps the person on this earth I am most grateful for is my wife of almost 35 years. Lora, you are incredible. You may not have had much to do with this manual, but you have everything to do with me. Without you I am not the same. The love, encouragement, wisdom and enjoyment you bring me is epic.

Yes, *literally* epic!

TABLE OF CONTENTS

The Starting Line

Welcome to the starting line! You're ready to tackle the race of life, which is an ultra-marathon with gusto, wisdom and joy! My hope for you is that you will excel as you have never excelled before and that you would pass on all that you learn in this process to others.

Just beginning this manual means you have set yourself up for success like you have never known it before. For so many of us, life is filled with passivity. It's like we wake up each day and wonder what is going to happen to us. We know we have to go to work or get the kids to school, we know we have to fulfill certain tasks throughout the day, but we let life take us by the hand and lead us. No successful person lives that way. From professional athletes to scientists, from straight-A students to CEOs, they all have one thing in common: they take the bull by the horns every day. They plan and purpose themselves to do the things that make them successful or at least create the opportunity for success. The same is true for marriages, finances, health and every area of life. If you want to excel, you have to be intentional. That is what the *TLP Life Manuals* are full of – intentionality.

There is something about you. You're different. You want it. You are willing to go after it. You have your sights set on something and want to attain it, or maybe you are tired of the same routine. You are tired of mediocre, or maybe you are just stuck in a certain place in life. You have decided that life should be lived to its fullest potential and it is starting *right now*. You want to live remarkably. Not only do you want to, you are actually doing something in order to live more remarkably. This manual is a starting place. Welcome to your next level!

The *TLP Life Manuals* are built upon honest evaluations and self-determination towards living a more remarkable life. If this becomes rote—a simple task to check off your to-do list—you are cutting its legs off. These manuals are meant to challenge you. I have provided the tools for the challenge, for honest assessments, and for a rocket-propelled future, but it is up to you to go after it like a hungry lion. You have what it takes!

It is important to note that you may discover things in your life while going through this process that are difficult to confront or difficult to overcome because of many factors, including deep emotional wounds. These things sometimes stunt our growth and without working through those issues, we can get stuck. I encourage you to be proactive if you find yourself in that situation. We all need help from time to time to get through difficult things. Maybe you can talk to a wise friend or a mentor. Mentors are minimized in our culture for various reasons. I find them very helpful to push over roadblocks. You may want to enlist the help of a pastor or a counselor for help as well. Whoever you choose, make sure they are dedicated to helping you get you through it and don't just name you by the trauma or wound you experienced. You can overcome your situation. God is for you! Although your past has an influence on your present, that is not your identity. Don't let your past limit you.

Total Life Pursuit Philosophy

Everything in you, or everything that makes up who you are, is connected. Everything about you affects everything else about you to some degree or another. We have tried our best to compartmentalize the different areas of our lives, but it isn't working. We bury things from our childhood, we bury things that happened yesterday and we think it doesn't affect us. Wrong! I am not trying to get everyone to go to counseling and talk about their childhood, but I am purporting that we cannot successfully compartmentalize our lives without a negative effect.

I heard of a guy who is a great dad, a good friend, served in the church, and loved God, yet separated his business life. To him, they just didn't go together. Unfortunately, it caught up with him and he suffered terribly for it. I have seen people's work-life ruin their marriage and I have also seen past emotional issues ruin their marriages and their work life. Even though this manual is singular in purpose, our life is *not* singular. It is plural. Just like we are spirit, soul and body, we have different areas of our life that overlap into each other.

The River Concept

The Mississippi River is a great example of this principle. Its main water source is Lake Itasca. It is also fed by small rivers like the Big Muddy River. It is then joined with other larger rivers along the way to the Gulf of Mexico, like the Missouri River. However, the Mississippi River feeds dozens of creeks, rivers, and lakes with the massive amount of water that it contains. We are like this in a way. The six major areas of life all feed each other and they all branch off from each other similar to the Mississippi River.

Let's look at the mental area of life, for example. It is fed by the spiritual, physical, relational, financial and emotional areas of life. Likewise, the mental area also feeds the spiritual, physical, relational, financial and emotional areas. They all interconnect. We are integrated and therefore compartmentalization always causes some kind of *dam* in our lives and restricts the full amount of life-giving flow to the other areas of our life. Let's say you have automatic negative thoughts (ANT's), running through your brain. Those negative thoughts affect your biochemistry which is your physical make-up. That affects your body which in turn affects your ability to think straight. Being negative can affect your relationships and it certainly can affect your ability to be in complete control of your emotions. That may send you to a counselor that you have to pay for, or more serious consequences like a physical disease caused by constant high stress.

The Six Major Areas

I hope you have become well acquainted with the six major areas of life by reading my first book, *Total Life Pursuit*. Each of the six areas has its own manual with the purpose of helping you become a better rendition of you, to help you grow, or as I like to put it, "raise you up a level in each individual area." I encourage you to work through every one of them like you are at stair one of the ground floor. If you are actually on the fourth floor you will get back to that level quickly, but if the first floor is your starting place, you will avoid overestimating yourself and missing some important basics. Here are the thrusts of each manual:

- *TLP Starting Line: Life Planning Manual* (in print) – Developing a mission, vision and plan for your life.
- *TLP Physical: Health Training Manual* (in print) – Becoming healthy and fit in your physical body through my four pillars of physical health.
- *TLP Spiritual Manual* (coming soon) – Define your core beliefs. Relate on a personal level with God.
- *TLP Mental & Emotional Manual* (coming soon) – Understand the deadly emotions and toxic thinking at play in your life in order to release you from their negative effects and constant stress. You will learn to create a positive mindset, eliminate stressors, grow your brain power and ultimately heal your soul so you can live in freedom from emotional rule.
- *TLP Relational Manual* (coming soon) – Bring health, vitality and real love to your relationships.
- *TLP Financial Manual* (coming soon) – Evaluate your finances. Create a plan to meet your stated goals.

At the end of most of the manuals, you will find a Life Goals section to help you develop short-term and long-term goals to meet for each manual's focus. You can return to any manual at any time to go deeper and work on achieving a new, higher level of living.

I urge you to complete all of the manuals on paper. There is something about writing and seeing it that cannot be duplicated on a device. I am a person that has my library on Kindle and my calendar synced across all my devices, however, when I do this each year, I write. I believe it is a must.

Each manual is designed to take 30-45 days. Some of the sections you will be able to finish quicker and other sections you may want to take longer to complete. Remember, this never ends, so you may copy the worksheet pages that are reproducible (labeled "reproducible by permission" at the bottom of the page) for personal use and use them again and again. Copy them, customize them, do what you need to for yourself in order to continue growing in these areas.

There are plenty of cool apps out there that will be helpful. However, be careful to avoid missing the big picture. A "To-Do" or "Task" list is great on your phone, but it is wise to see a daily, weekly and monthly view. Also, you will need lists for objectives and projects as well as your tasks. Choose wisely after you do it on paper.

In order to fully plan, you will also need to know your destination. Remember what I said about passively going throughout your day(s)? If you want to get to a destination you have to go in that direction. There is something that is at your core. It is your purpose. What is your life mission? It is funny how hard that can be to articulate. This manual will help you produce a well thought out life mission statement. It is absolutely freeing when you have an understanding of what you are supposed to do with your life.

So many are afraid to write their goals down for fear of not attaining them. That's not you! You are not like that. You are afraid of nothing. You write down goals and celebrate each step you make toward them. For the goals you don't attain by the time you had planned, schedule it again and conquer that hill with no guilt to persuade you otherwise.

Purpose of this Manual

This is not a class workbook, nor something to finish (as in you start it just to finish it). Certainly you are a finisher and you will finish everything you start unless you make the conscious decision not to for some reason. This is not a workbook that goes along with my book, *Total Life Pursuit,* that should be used side by side. This is a life-changing, self-paced manual to help plan your life with intentionality where you will go deep, make necessary choices, mobilize your strength, and use effort to see the change that you want to see. Whether you are going through this solo, with another person, or with a group, don't let yourself slip into the, "I've gotta' get it done," approach where you are answering questions as fast as possible to complete your assignment. You will get out of this what you put into it. Enjoy the process. Take your time. Set up a daily appointment with yourself. You are worth it and it will pay more dividends than most things you do. Nearly every successful person in life has personal development time built into their life. You are that person now. Put this time in your schedule. Also, invite God into the process since He is for your success! Talk to Him. Ask Him questions. Ask him to guide your mind, brain and heart. Put in your strength, effort and a concrete series of choices and you will see great changes. (And so will everyone else.)

Your Approach

You can't focus on every area of life at once. You do have to pick a starting place. Whether this manual is the first one you are doing or the last, it will benefit you beyond what you think. However, if it is the first like I hope it is, perform this quick exercise and learn some valuable insights about where to start.

What area do I think I need the most work in? _____

Why do I think I need the most work in this area?

_____

_____

_____

What would my closest friend say I should start with? (Write the answer and then ask them!)

_____

What did they say? _____

What area am I most passionate about? _____

What area would I like to avoid? _____

What area would be most beneficial for me to grow in, and to others around me?

_____

What area would best benefit the other areas, and therefore my life? _____

Do you have a picture of what you need to work on yet? After this manual, start there. I believe that if you get your schedule aligned with who you are and what you are on this earth to do, then you will better be able to implement the choices that you have made. You will know how to adjust your schedule accordingly. Maybe there is no time for assessing your finances, because you never do. You can come back to the schedule that you have done in this manual and alter it. You may find yourself finding new purpose or place things at a higher or lower priority in your life, then come back to these exercises and see if they are still accurate. Many things in this manual are moving, shifting, changing and elevating. That is why you would be wise to do what you will do here every year.

Honesty

Throughout this manual are deep, sometimes heart-pounding questions that will challenge the most authentic of us. They will pry your heart open if you will let them. They need to be thought through in order to have the desired effect. That takes honesty.

I have a scale that I bring out at our church gym, Total Fit Gym. This scale measures weight but also, through an algorithm and electrical impedance, your body fat percentage. It is amazing how many people don't want to know. I always ask them why not, why don't you want to know? They almost always say, I know my fat percentage is high and I don't want to know the number. You may be like that too. That's okay, for now, but let's look at this a little closer. Maybe you are heavier than you want to be, maybe than you should be, and you know it. Okay, that is scary, but you already know it, right? Are you with me? You know it, so the scale is only going to confirm what you already know. So if you step on the scale you will see it with your eyes. Maybe there is something inside of you that is hoping what you know isn't true? Like the person who thinks their bank account balance is $1000.00 at the end of the month. They haven't balanced their books, but that is a good estimation. They want to purchase an item that costs $1500.00, so they hope what they know is wrong and they go ahead and buy it. Are you tracking with me? The man who thinks his marriage is just fine, but the wife wants to go to marriage counseling, but he won't go. Why? Because he really doesn't think it is just fine. In fact, he is afraid of finding out exactly what he knows, the marriage is in trouble. What is the preoccupation with not knowing, or seeing the truth? Why not?

Before you read on, complete this statement: I sometimes don't want to see the truth because...

_____

_____

_____

_____

There is a woman that we will call Sally. She looked at the scale and flat out refused to step on it. Sally is beautiful. Her body is fantastic. Many women would be jealous of her figure. She probably has gained 5-10 pounds more than she likes. In her mind she is fat. She doesn't want to know how fat. If she would just get on the scale she would actually find out that she is less fat than she thinks!

There is another woman and her real name is Cassandra (a real woman - her name is used with permission). She is a little over halfway to her goal of losing 100 pounds. She has more fat than Sally but she doesn't hesitate to get on the scale. When I gave her a high five and told her I was proud of her she said, "It's not like this fat is staying." Did you get that? Her present condition did NOT define her. She knew that she was on her way to her goal so she didn't value the number that the scale would give her as her forever spot in life. She saw it as a *tool* to measure her *progress*. Please notice the words *tools* and *progress*. That is what evaluations are; they are tools to help understand where you are in your progress...your thinking, your weight, your marriage or whatever else. Evaluations of these areas are done as progress trackers.

Without proper and honest evaluations, you will be hindered from reaching your potential or even your next level in any area. If you think you are just fine then you won't reach higher. If you are afraid of knowing the truth, you already believe some kind of lie and you need to find out what lie you believe so you can get rid of that thinking. If you never evaluate where you are, you will never be able to fully celebrate your progress. The questions may be penetrating and uncomfortable, but so what? Greatness is waiting.

Change

Choice + Strength + Effort = Change

Your life has certain inertia, and if you are going to change it will take more effort to change than to remain the same. To change the inertia of an object takes more energy. To excel in anything takes personal responsibility and requisitioning the strength within you. The good news is that you have the strength and determination that it takes! Here are the mechanics and steps to change.

Step 1: Decide, choose to go for it! It is one of the most powerful things in your being. You get to choose. Keep it real. Dream big, but keep it within the realm of possibility in your head. You are the one that has to believe it is attainable.

Do it right now with a financial goal. What have you decided? Detail it a little.

_____

_____

_____

Step 2: Envision the next level. You not only have to envision your end goal, but you have to envision the *next level*. What does it look like? How do you behave to attain it? How do you behave after you attain it? How do you feel having attained it? Not your end game, just the next step. Write it down. Look at it regularly.

Write a physical goal down here. What is your first level goal? Not your end goal, just your first milestone. (i.e., *My goal is to lose 30 pounds. My first milestone is to lose two pounds.*)

Goal: _____

First milestone: _____

Step 3: Plan it. Schedule it. Purpose it. Count the cost. See the benefit! You have to put whatever you are going to do in your schedule. (That's why I like people to start with this manual). So count the cost and weigh it against the benefit before you start. Be convinced that it is worthwhile.

At what time will you work through the manual every day? _____ Now put it in your phone or calendar with a pop up reminder.

Step 4: Get a tool to track your successes. The tool may be a tape measure (I advise against scales as your physical evaluation tool – weight is deceiving when you are building muscle), a friend's assessment, money in your bank account, or feeling less stressed.

For this manual, what tools will you use to evaluate your progress?

_____

_____

_____

Step 5: Be in community. If applicable, find a group or a couple of friends that are like-minded that have similar types of goals. You could always start a group yourself.

As you work on this manual, name someone you can get to be on your team, to hold you accountable to growth

in this area? _____

Step 6: Do it! Get in motion! Get your foot on the gas, put it in first gear and get going.

What is your first step for getting to the next level? What will you do today or tomorrow?

_____

_____

_____

_____

Are you ready to go? You have more control than you think. How you think is so important. Thinking a loving thought relaxes your DNA within 30 seconds.[1] Thinking a hateful thought tightens your DNA within 30 seconds. You have so much power, so much control. Don't ever be convinced that you are trapped. You are not. God is for you—He wants the best for you!

Solomon, the wisest man and probably the richest man on earth said something important about our thoughts. I believe that it was God who spoke through him when he said, "The tongue has the power of life and death." (Proverbs 18:21) He continued on to say, "those who love it will eat its fruit." Your tongue can produce fruit that is going to taste really good. There is this cycle that happens through our thinking, speaking and hearing that is so powerful. Get your mouth pointing you in the direction you want to go. It's not magic, but it is like the steering wheel of a vessel. It points you—and more.

---

[1]   Glen Rein, PhD, and Rollin McCraty, PhD, "Local and Non-Local Effects of Coherent Heart Frequencies on Conformational Changes of DNA," Institute of HeartMath, January 1, 2011, http://appreciativeinquiry.case.edu/practice/organizationDetail.cfm?coid=852&sector=32, accessed October 5, 2013.

Smart Goals

Smart is an acronym I want you to remember when you create all of your goals. Every goal must be run through this matrix. You may find that a few goals can't be measured by this, but the vast majority must be.

Specific – Create goals that are detailed and specific. Something you can throw a dart at and hit the bull's eye. (i.e., I will read one book per month).

Measurable – The goal has to have a measure so you can see if you have attained it and then celebrate the win! (i.e., I will lose three inches off my waistline vs. I want to lose weight from my waistline).

Attainable – The goal must be attainable. It has to be realistic. You have to be able to get a "W" (win) for achieving it. (i.e., I will go on a date with my spouse once a week).

Relevant – The goal must be relevant and applicable to the specific thing you are trying to attain. (i.e., if you are trying to save your income for an emergency fund, the goal must be specific to saving money, spending practices or income generation).

Time-bound – The goal must be tied to a time frame or specific date for completion. (i.e., I am going to express forgiveness to my mom for being an alcoholic during my childhood in the next two weeks).

Basic Goals

Life Planning

I want my life to have more: _____

If I could change one thing about the way my daily life flows it would be: _____
_____

Anytime I think about or am asked about my goals, the top three things I think about are:

1. _____

2. _____

3. _____

Because I want you to keep in mind all six areas of life as you go through this manual, I would like you to write your responses to the following questions.

Spiritual

Name two goals that would propel you in this area of life.

1. _____

2. _____

Physical

Name up to three goals that can be attained in eight weeks that you can break down into smaller weekly goals.

1. _____

2. _____

3. _____

Mental

List three goals that would help you live life with maximum enjoyment.

1. _____

2. _____

3. _____

Emotional

Name one goal to reduce your stress level and one toxic emotion that you would like to remove from your life.

1. _____

2. _____

Relational

List one thing you need to work on in regards to interpersonal relationships.

_____

If you are married, list one goal for your marriage. If you are single, list one goal that will prepare you to be a great spouse.

_____

Financial

Name two financial goals that you can attain within six months:

1. _____

2. _____

Total Life

The top three things I want to change about my life are:

1. _____

2. _____

3. _____

The number one thing I need to change about my life is:

_____

The most important area of life I need to change that will most affect the other areas is:

_____

Life Planning

There are people who are driven through life and then there are the drivers. The principles in this chapter will make you a driver. When you are the driver you get to go where you want to most of the time. There will always be things that pop up in your life that are unexpected or that you can't plan for, but your life direction will continue to go where you want it to. Every chapter is exciting and every chapter will challenge you. This chapter, however, will position you for success in every area of life.

CEOs and other movers and shakers have assistants. One of the reasons they have assistants is to remove them from the smaller tasks of their position and even their personal lives. The other reason, and possibly the number one thing a good assistant can do, is to organize your schedule and keep you on task. Assistants are one of the most important positions in a company because they keep one of the most important people in the company focused on the most important things in order to keep the company profitable and growing. Unfortunately, most of us don't have assistants. We are the CEOs, CAOs, CFOs and all of their assistants of our own lives. Maybe you are lucky enough to have a spouse that fills that role, but for most of us, the spouse is also a CEO, CAO or CFO and they too need an assistant!

CEOs didn't always have assistants. They started out ruling their own schedules and making decisions that would put them in a position for advancement. They decided what would fill their day and it probably wasn't checking Instagram or Facebook. They created priorities based on their mission, and those priorities became their "big rocks" that would dominate their schedule and produce the results that helped them rise to CEO status. My postulation is all of us are CEOs of one thing or another and we need to start acting like it. There is much more to life than business. There is marriage, parenting, homemaking, your relationship with God, volunteer work, friendships, hobbies, education, financial engineering, landscaping, purchasing, and a dozen more things to fill your days. I didn't even mention social media which, you know, can't be understated! We have things pulling at us, including our TVs, in every direction. We have offers to do this or do that, and we only have so much of the most valuable resource on God's green earth. Time!

How you will spend your weeks, days and hours has got to be determined ahead of time for the most part. I am not talking about determining it at the beginning of the day, I am saying we need to, at the beginning of the year fashion our daily outlook. Some of you don't like to schedule. You may feel resistance to do any of the following exercises. You are thinking you should skip this chapter. You have never scheduled your life and it is going just fine. My challenge to you is to try it for a couple of months. If you don't see an improvement, then switch back and fly by the seat of your pants. If, however, you do see improvement, go back and work through this chapter thoroughly, then drop me a thank you email.

Before we do anything, let's see if you can come up with some time wasters in your life. Not necessarily the things that you find enjoyment and relaxation doing, but things that keep you from the more important things of life. See if you can name ten time wasters in your life.

1. _____

2. _____

3. _____

4. _____

5. _____

6. _____

7. _____

8. _____

9. _____

10. _____

Now go back through them and write a number value next to them based on which ones waste the most cumulative time (e.g., internet surfing = 10, because it wastes the most time).

Now fill in this chart:

Time waster	Time per occurrence	Occurrences per day	Daily time	Weekly time	Monthly time

Here is another tool for tracking how much time you spend on things. We often do not realize how much time we spend on the internet "dorking" around. Okay, clothes shopping isn't "dorking," right? And neither is Facebook or Instagram!? Let's get honest here. I have included a media journal to help. For the next week, log any type of media use that totals more than five minutes. Yes, that includes your phone. In fact, there is a great feature on most phones that tracks your screen time and what apps are being used. Use it. Then write down the week's summation.

Media Journal

Date	Show / Internet	Time Spent
Jan 11	*Reality T.V. (Example)*	*1 hr*
Jan 11	*YouTube (Example)*	*30 mins*

Media Journal

Date	Show / Internet	Time Spent

Media Journal

Date	Show / Internet	Time Spent

Media Journal

Date	Show / Internet	Time Spent

<u>Weekly Summary</u>

Record the total time from your Media Journal by category:

Social Media	Television	Internet browsing	Idle online shopping	Other	Other

How did you do? Write your observations below.

_____

_____

_____

_____

What needs to change?

_____

_____

_____

_____

How will you accomplish change? What specific measures will you use to get to where you want to be?

_____

_____

_____

_____

Time Tracking

One of the interesting things you can do to see where your time goes at work, even if your home is your work, is to track your time. How much time do you spend on answering emails, creativity, administrating basic functions of your job or communicating with team members? It comes in handy, especially if you are honest enough to list all the time you waste. It is no secret that employees can waste several hours a day on non-job related surfing, texting, and social media use. If you're a manager, it may be useful to track your team's time in order to assess the value of certain activities. If you are self-employed, this is a must. You have to know where your time is going. If you are a stay-at-home wife/husband or mom/dad, and have the jobs of a dozen people. I would challenge you to track your time as well. Your efficiency is just as important as any CEO. Everyone should remember that some downtime during the day is a wonderful thing. When I do this exercise I am proud to have some spaces in my day where I do nothing.

There are many apps out there that track your time with an ongoing clock. Most of them have a paid subscription. If you have an iPhone or Android, you can easily track your screen time. It may be very insightful, but first, you will have to overcome your fear of what you will see. However, screen time is not what we are after. You want to see where your time is actually going in all areas. You may continue to work through this workbook, but I encourage you to log your time on these worksheets. When you are done with the week, study it and take notes of the good, bad and the ugly.

Time	Activity	Time	Activity
6:00 am		2:00 pm	
6:15 am		2:15 pm	
6:30 am		2:30 pm	
6:45 am		2:45 pm	
7:00 am		3:00 pm	
7:15 am		3:15 pm	
7:30 am		3:30 pm	
7:45 am		3:45 pm	
8:00 am		4:00 pm	
8:15 am		4:15 pm	
8:30 am		4:30 pm	
8:45 am		4:45 pm	
9:00 am		5:00 pm	
9:15 am		5:15 pm	
9:30 am		5:30 pm	
9:45 am		5:45 pm	
10:00 am		6:00 pm	
10:15 am		6:15 pm	
10:30 am		6:30 pm	
10:45 am		6:45 pm	
11:00 am		7:00 pm	
11:15 am		7:15 pm	
11:30 am		7:30 pm	
11:45 am		7:45 pm	
12:00 pm		8:00 pm	
12:15 pm		8:15 pm	
12:30 pm		8:30 pm	
12:45 pm		8:45 pm	
1:00 pm		9:00 pm	
1:15 pm		9:15 pm	
1:30 pm		9:30 pm	
1:45 pm		9:45 pm	

Time	Activity	Time	Activity
6:00 am		2:00 pm	
6:15 am		2:15 pm	
6:30 am		2:30 pm	
6:45 am		2:45 pm	
7:00 am		3:00 pm	
7:15 am		3:15 pm	
7:30 am		3:30 pm	
7:45 am		3:45 pm	
8:00 am		4:00 pm	
8:15 am		4:15 pm	
8:30 am		4:30 pm	
8:45 am		4:45 pm	
9:00 am		5:00 pm	
9:15 am		5:15 pm	
9:30 am		5:30 pm	
9:45 am		5:45 pm	
10:00 am		6:00 pm	
10:15 am		6:15 pm	
10:30 am		6:30 pm	
10:45 am		6:45 pm	
11:00 am		7:00 pm	
11:15 am		7:15 pm	
11:30 am		7:30 pm	
11:45 am		7:45 pm	
12:00 pm		8:00 pm	
12:15 pm		8:15 pm	
12:30 pm		8:30 pm	
12:45 pm		8:45 pm	
1:00 pm		9:00 pm	
1:15 pm		9:15 pm	
1:30 pm		9:30 pm	
1:45 pm		9:45 pm	

Time	Activity	Time	Activity
6:00 am		2:00 pm	
6:15 am		2:15 pm	
6:30 am		2:30 pm	
6:45 am		2:45 pm	
7:00 am		3:00 pm	
7:15 am		3:15 pm	
7:30 am		3:30 pm	
7:45 am		3:45 pm	
8:00 am		4:00 pm	
8:15 am		4:15 pm	
8:30 am		4:30 pm	
8:45 am		4:45 pm	
9:00 am		5:00 pm	
9:15 am		5:15 pm	
9:30 am		5:30 pm	
9:45 am		5:45 pm	
10:00 am		6:00 pm	
10:15 am		6:15 pm	
10:30 am		6:30 pm	
10:45 am		6:45 pm	
11:00 am		7:00 pm	
11:15 am		7:15 pm	
11:30 am		7:30 pm	
11:45 am		7:45 pm	
12:00 pm		8:00 pm	
12:15 pm		8:15 pm	
12:30 pm		8:30 pm	
12:45 pm		8:45 pm	
1:00 pm		9:00 pm	
1:15 pm		9:15 pm	
1:30 pm		9:30 pm	
1:45 pm		9:45 pm	

Time	Activity	Time	Activity
6:00 am		2:00 pm	
6:15 am		2:15 pm	
6:30 am		2:30 pm	
6:45 am		2:45 pm	
7:00 am		3:00 pm	
7:15 am		3:15 pm	
7:30 am		3:30 pm	
7:45 am		3:45 pm	
8:00 am		4:00 pm	
8:15 am		4:15 pm	
8:30 am		4:30 pm	
8:45 am		4:45 pm	
9:00 am		5:00 pm	
9:15 am		5:15 pm	
9:30 am		5:30 pm	
9:45 am		5:45 pm	
10:00 am		6:00 pm	
10:15 am		6:15 pm	
10:30 am		6:30 pm	
10:45 am		6:45 pm	
11:00 am		7:00 pm	
11:15 am		7:15 pm	
11:30 am		7:30 pm	
11:45 am		7:45 pm	
12:00 pm		8:00 pm	
12:15 pm		8:15 pm	
12:30 pm		8:30 pm	
12:45 pm		8:45 pm	
1:00 pm		9:00 pm	
1:15 pm		9:15 pm	
1:30 pm		9:30 pm	
1:45 pm		9:45 pm	

Time	Activity	Time	Activity
6:00 am		2:00 pm	
6:15 am		2:15 pm	
6:30 am		2:30 pm	
6:45 am		2:45 pm	
7:00 am		3:00 pm	
7:15 am		3:15 pm	
7:30 am		3:30 pm	
7:45 am		3:45 pm	
8:00 am		4:00 pm	
8:15 am		4:15 pm	
8:30 am		4:30 pm	
8:45 am		4:45 pm	
9:00 am		5:00 pm	
9:15 am		5:15 pm	
9:30 am		5:30 pm	
9:45 am		5:45 pm	
10:00 am		6:00 pm	
10:15 am		6:15 pm	
10:30 am		6:30 pm	
10:45 am		6:45 pm	
11:00 am		7:00 pm	
11:15 am		7:15 pm	
11:30 am		7:30 pm	
11:45 am		7:45 pm	
12:00 pm		8:00 pm	
12:15 pm		8:15 pm	
12:30 pm		8:30 pm	
12:45 pm		8:45 pm	
1:00 pm		9:00 pm	
1:15 pm		9:15 pm	
1:30 pm		9:30 pm	
1:45 pm		9:45 pm	

Time	Activity	Time	Activity
6:00 am		2:00 pm	
6:15 am		2:15 pm	
6:30 am		2:30 pm	
6:45 am		2:45 pm	
7:00 am		3:00 pm	
7:15 am		3:15 pm	
7:30 am		3:30 pm	
7:45 am		3:45 pm	
8:00 am		4:00 pm	
8:15 am		4:15 pm	
8:30 am		4:30 pm	
8:45 am		4:45 pm	
9:00 am		5:00 pm	
9:15 am		5:15 pm	
9:30 am		5:30 pm	
9:45 am		5:45 pm	
10:00 am		6:00 pm	
10:15 am		6:15 pm	
10:30 am		6:30 pm	
10:45 am		6:45 pm	
11:00 am		7:00 pm	
11:15 am		7:15 pm	
11:30 am		7:30 pm	
11:45 am		7:45 pm	
12:00 pm		8:00 pm	
12:15 pm		8:15 pm	
12:30 pm		8:30 pm	
12:45 pm		8:45 pm	
1:00 pm		9:00 pm	
1:15 pm		9:15 pm	
1:30 pm		9:30 pm	
1:45 pm		9:45 pm	

Time	Activity	Time	Activity
6:00 am		2:00 pm	
6:15 am		2:15 pm	
6:30 am		2:30 pm	
6:45 am		2:45 pm	
7:00 am		3:00 pm	
7:15 am		3:15 pm	
7:30 am		3:30 pm	
7:45 am		3:45 pm	
8:00 am		4:00 pm	
8:15 am		4:15 pm	
8:30 am		4:30 pm	
8:45 am		4:45 pm	
9:00 am		5:00 pm	
9:15 am		5:15 pm	
9:30 am		5:30 pm	
9:45 am		5:45 pm	
10:00 am		6:00 pm	
10:15 am		6:15 pm	
10:30 am		6:30 pm	
10:45 am		6:45 pm	
11:00 am		7:00 pm	
11:15 am		7:15 pm	
11:30 am		7:30 pm	
11:45 am		7:45 pm	
12:00 pm		8:00 pm	
12:15 pm		8:15 pm	
12:30 pm		8:30 pm	
12:45 pm		8:45 pm	
1:00 pm		9:00 pm	
1:15 pm		9:15 pm	
1:30 pm		9:30 pm	
1:45 pm		9:45 pm	

How did you do? What did you find out that amazed you?

_____

_____

_____

_____

_____

What do you need to cut down or cut out?

_____

_____

_____

_____

_____

What were you happy to find?

_____

_____

_____

_____

_____

You are now ready to tackle the number one priority, the understanding of and defining your mission. It is your mission that will ultimately help you set your daily agenda and your goals for the day, week, month, year and beyond. You have already created goals in a previous section, but those goals are not what defines your mission. Your mission defines your goals. I included that section to get you to think about your future. You may find at the end of this exercise that those goals accurately reflect your mission, or you may find that you create new goals that better align with your stated mission. Either way, I encourage you to not go back and look at those goals until you are done with this manual. Now is your time to define your life mission. Be thoughtful.

Mission

If I asked you to tell me the top two most important things that you do, and I gave you 30 seconds to answer, what would the answers be? Go! You have 30 seconds to write:

1. _____

2. _____

If you had one day left to live and I asked you to tell me the top two most important things you have accomplished in life so far, what would your answer be?

1. _____

2. _____

If you asked God what the top three things you were made for are, what do you think He would say?

1. _____

2. _____

3. _____

The first step to any type of plan, whether it is a business plan or a life plan, is to find your mission. There are many ways to define mission, but for our purposes your mission is your purpose in life. It is the place you want to be—a defined destination. It isn't so much about who you are, it is more about where you are going. For instance, two of my missions in life are to be a great husband and to be a great father. I *am* a husband and I *am* a father, but my mission is to actually do the things it takes to be great in each of these roles. If I am honest with myself, I can self-assess and see if I am staying true to these missions. We all have several missions that will guide our lives if we take the time to articulate them in writing. At the end of this section, I will ask you to boil down your different missions into one overarching mission statement. When you write this big picture mission it can get difficult to convey and it becomes more of a process than you first thought. That is a good thing. This is your life mission! It will direct your course for decades to come.

Mission Exercise

So many people go through life without a true compass to direct them to where they want to end up. They get a job, get a spouse, have some kids, buy a house and look forward to retirement. Those aren't bad, however, you have to have purpose in it. There has to be an end game to fuel you through the very long, and at times tough, game itself. Like an NFL team works hard toward winning a Super Bowl, it is incumbent upon us to develop a mission to guide us to our Super Bowl win! It is the mapped out course we sail that gets us to the correct destination.

Because each individual is unique, a personal mission statement will reflect that uniqueness, both in content and form. Writing an empowering mission statement is not a task to be checked off. To be empowering, it has to become a living document. It represents a lifetime balance of the personal, family, work, and community roles you fill. It is written to inspire *you*, not to impress anyone else.

Your mission must be written, clearly defined and understood. This may take some time. Be patient in the process. The favorable outcome of your life depends on it. What follows are many questions to get you thinking. Write down the answers to these questions and then begin to enlarge your thinking to incorporate all that your mission(s) may include.

Step 1: Identify Past Successes. Spend some time identifying four or five examples where you have had personal success in recent years. These successes could be at work, in your community, at home, etc. Write them down.

_____

_____

_____

_____

_____

_____

_____

_____

_____

_____

_____

_____

_____

_____

Try to identify whether there is a common theme(s) to these examples. Write them down.

_____

_____

_____

_____

Step 2: Identify Core Values. Develop a list of attributes that you believe identify what you value, who you are and what your priorities are. The list can be as long as you need. (E.g., Do you believe in honesty, justice, kindness, and self-reliance?)

_____

_____

_____

_____

_____

_____

_____

Go back and assign a number value to each core value listed and then list them in order beginning with the highest priority value.

_____

_____

_____

_____

_____

_____

_____

Go back through your list and see if you could best be described as a person who has only the top five values. Rearrange your list if need be.

1._____

2._____

3._____

4._____

5._____

Finally, see if your number one value is what other people would say you value most. (If you are daring, ask your best friend or spouse if they agree.)

My number one value: _____

Do others agree? _____

Step 3 – Reflect on your life. What is your inspiration? What do you love? What do you love about yourself? Who has inspired you?

_____

_____

_____

_____

_____

_____

_____

_____

_____

_____

_____

_____

_____

Do you want to have qualities similar to those folks? Figure out what those qualities are and list them.

_____

_____

_____

_____

_____

What big events impacted your life? They could be positive or negative. Reflect on these big moments and the lessons you learned from them.

_____

_____

_____

_____

Thinking about the negative things that impacted your life, can you identify any lingering negative effects? If so, write how it is still affecting you and what steps you could take to overcome those effects.

_____

_____

_____

_____

_____

What do you love about your life? Your work? Your family, friends, and other relationships?

_____

_____

_____

_____

_____

_____

_____

When are you at your best? What do you have the talent to do really well?

_____

_____

_____

_____

_____

_____

_____

_____

When are you at your worst?

_____

_____

_____

_____

_____

_____

_____

_____

What would you like to improve about yourself?

_____

_____

_____

_____

_____

_____

_____

What would you like to share with others? What talents and abilities can you give to your community?

_____

_____

_____

_____

_____

_____

_____

What things do you want to pass down to your children/grandchildren? (Whether you have them or not)

_____

_____

_____

_____

_____

_____

_____

If you had unlimited resources and unlimited time, what would you choose to do?

_____

_____

_____

_____

_____

_____

_____

_____

What are your greatest strengths?

_____

_____

_____

_____

_____

_____

_____

_____

_____

_____

What are the three or four most important things to you in life?

_____

_____

_____

_____

_____

_____

_____

_____

_____

How do you want to be remembered?

_____

_____

_____

_____

_____

_____

_____

_____

Step 4: Identify Your Heart. Make a list of the ways you could and would like to make a difference. In an ideal situation, how could you contribute best to:

Your family:

_____

_____

_____

_____

_____

_____

_____

_____

Your friends:

_____

_____

_____

_____

_____

_____

_____

_____

Your community:

_____

_____

_____

_____

_____

_____

_____

_____

Your employer or future employers:

_____

_____

_____

_____

_____

_____

_____

_____

_____

Your church:

_____

_____

_____

_____

_____

_____

_____

_____

_____

The world in general:

_____

_____

_____

_____

_____

_____

_____

_____

Step 5: Identify Goals. Spend some time thinking about your priorities in life and the goals you have for yourself.

Make a list of your personal goals in the six major areas of life. (Do not use the goals you wrote in the beginning of this manual. Let yourself be guided by God and by what you have already discovered and written about yourself).

Spiritual: _____

_____

_____

_____

Mental: _____

_____

_____

_____

Physical: _____

_____

_____

_____

Emotional: _____

_____

_____

_____

Relational: _____

_____

_____

_____

Financial: _____

_____

_____

_____

General life goals: _____

_____

_____

_____

_____

_____

_____

_____

_____

_____

Step 6: Write Your Mission Statement. Based on the first five steps and a better understanding of yourself, begin writing your personal mission statement (3-5 sentences long).

Say what you want to have happen, don't speak in the negative. If at the end of your life people wrote tribute statements about the difference you have made in their life, what would you want to be said? That needs to be in this statement. Fill it with passion. Something you want to show your close friends and family. Something that will guide you day by day. Make it clear enough that if other people were to read it, they would instantly understand what you mean.

If you are really struggling to conceptualize this, read no more than five mission statements of companies or groups. What I want you to be able to do is understand what a mission statement looks like, but I want you to completely create your own. Do not read any personal mission statements.

_____

_____

_____

_____

_____

_____

_____

_____

_____

_____

_____

_____

Next is perhaps the most difficult thing. *I want you to boil these 3-5 sentences down to one sentence or just a phrase.* I know this is difficult because I have done it many times. To help, write your long mission statement down on your phone or a sticky note some place where you will see if often. You have to get at the essence of your personal mission in life. Go for it. Take some time to think it through. Try writing down your ideas so you can see them. Put them on a whiteboard or sticky notes and pretend you are coming up with the next big campaign for a new product. Dial it in. Come back to it often until you have nailed it down.

_____

_____

_____

_____

Now try to boil it down to a phrase or a few words that would explain the basic concept of your vision to a stranger.

Your mission statement:

_____

If the above sentence is more than 15-20 words, do it again! I know it is easier to take the 3-5 sentences and make one long run-on sentence, but this needs to be concise. If necessary, rewrite it again. You are almost there. Don't give up.

The Four Quadrant Approach

There is a popular quadrant approach created by Stephen Covey (shown below). It illustrates how to schedule yourself for success. You can read about this in depth in many books and websites, including mine. There are four quadrants that we operate in.[2]

Quadrant I: Urgent & Important	Quadrant II: Not Urgent & Important
Quadrant III: Urgent & Not Important	Quadrant IV: Not Urgent & Not Important

Quadrant I is for the immediate and important deadlines.

Quadrant II is for long-term strategizing and development.

Quadrant III is for time-pressured distractions. They are not really important, but someone wants it now.

Quadrant IV is for those activities that yield little in any value. These are activities that are often used for taking a break in time-pressured and important activities.

The one thing we all do not want to do is live under the tyranny of the urgent. Tyranny of any kind is prohibitive for a life of freedom, especially the urgent! In our society this is ever-increasing with busy/hurry sickness, we can easily find ourselves in the middle of the "time crunch" that never ends. Some of us like operating here. We like the adrenaline or we like feeling the pressure, or maybe we get a boost in our significance if things are depending on our immediate intervention. Whatever the thinking, first we have to discover which quadrant we like most and which quadrant we operate in most. Dumping or delegating our tasks is very helpful, however, if the mental urge to be in a hurry isn't addressed, we will forever be slaves to the tyranny of the urgent.

The first quadrant keeps you on the mouse wheel, the third keeps you distracted, the fourth ruins you and the second is where you want to spend your time. The important stuff. The hope is you will concentrate on the important stuff all the time so rarely do you have any urgent things come across your desk because you have already taken care of them.

The following questions will help you discover where you operate now?

Do you feel under pressure to complete certain tasks or projects during most days? Explain.

_____

_____

_____

_____

[2]   http://www.visionstoexcellence.com/stephen-covey-4-quadrants/

What percentage of your day is spent under pressure to fulfill your responsibilites?

_____

If I was asking your parent, spouse or best friend, would they say you are a procrastinator?

_____

Is your normal operational mode to be in a hurry? Explain.

_____

_____

_____

_____

_____

When a project is on time and everything is being completed wonderfully, do you still stress out?

_____

_____

Do you create drama when everything is going great? (Think long and hard about this one.)

_____

_____

_____

_____

_____

Do you create inner turmoil when it isn't necessary? (Think deep about this and answer honestly.)

_____

_____

_____

Does drama seem to find you? Do you find yourself in situations that are contentious regularly? Explain.

_____

_____

_____

_____

_____

Do you like action and adventure movies more than all others?

_____

Do you seek peaceful times? If yes, explain how you seek those times?

_____

_____

_____

_____

_____

If yes, how successful are you at achieving a peaceful inner life?

_____

_____

_____

_____

_____

Are you a thrill seeker?

_____

_____

_____

Do you find that your close relationships are stable and without contention? Explain and use an example of the two closest relationships you have.

_____

_____

_____

_____

_____

_____

_____

_____

_____

It is important to self-assess so you can be self-aware. This is a skill that is learned. We learn to dodge and to hide and must concentrate in order to be brutally honest with ourselves. Go back over your answers and see if you would want to change anything. Then write down what you have learned. What quadrant(s) do you mainly operate in? Summarize it below like you are reading the answers that someone else has given.

_____

_____

_____

_____

_____

_____

_____

_____

_____

_____

_____

_____

_____

_____

_____

_____

In order to get out of the urgent and important quadrant, we must reject the NEED to be in the urgent. It is easy to fall into that rut. It can make us feel important. It can give us the adrenaline boost we like. The adrenal hormones can actually help us operate with laser focus. Sometimes we are just so behind on our schedule that we can't see our way out of the urgent and important quadrant hole. Hopefully, you have seen and can now address some issues with the way you operate by examining the answers to the above questions honestly. Now what? Change. It isn't easy, but it isn't too hard either. Some people have been operating this way their whole lives. Maybe that is you. Some people just get caught in this pattern because of circumstances outside of their control. Regardless of whether you chose this pattern or not, you need some help getting out.

In my *TLP Mental and Emotional Manual* is a program I have developed to help people rewrite their brains. Basically, you have to replace your current foundational thinking with a new thought. The steps involved and how to find the foundational thought(s) that are messing you up and hindering your progress is something I help you work through in the manual. The process is too long to insert here. My encouragement is to work through that manual after you complete this one.

Here are a few questions to help you get off the mouse wheel of the first, third or fourth quadrants.

What quadrant do you operate in most of your average day?

_____

Why is that?

_____

_____

_____

_____

_____

_____

_____

What quadrant do you operate in most of your week?

_____

What are the behaviors that keep you in the quadrants you don't want to be in?

_____

_____

_____

_____

_____

What are the foundational thought(s) that keeps you in the quadrant you don't want to be in?

_____

_____

_____

_____

_____

_____

_____

_____

_____

_____

_____

_____

If you had to boil it down to a belief statement that you have directing your life, what would it be? (E.g., I believe that I need to be busy to be important.)

_____

_____

_____

_____

_____

_____

_____

_____

_____

_____

Every great leader operates in Quadrant II, the not urgent but important quadrant a vast majority of the time. The tyranny of the urgent runs your life and as a taskmaster. You are better off living in the important things that aren't urgent. Sure, urgent things come up, however, when you plan and purpose your life, you are not caught in the urgent that much. In Quadrant II is where you must find your home. In the lower two quadrants, you can see that you, as the boss, can't spend your time with unimportant things. You must dump or delegate them. You are too important to spend your time on unimportant things. Sure, you can take a little break and get a little dopamine boost by accomplishing an easy task, however, if more than 5% of your time is in the not important quadrants, you will reduce your ability to control your destiny. You have a mission to accomplish. Your mission is important. Stick with that.

By answering the above questions, you may be able to see how to get yourself in the correct quadrant. Change your thinking. Change your core beliefs about your life, success, value and importance. As I said, I help you to do that in the *TLP Mental & Emotional Manual*. So for now, recognize the flaw of your thinking and keep working through the process in this manual. It will be beneficial if you plan better even if you haven't changed your core thoughts. Although, I plead with you to change your thinking. For now, keep working right here where you are. You will find yourself, at the completion of this journey, ready to tackle life the way you were purposed to.

Driving Your Life

Now let's take a look at how you are going to drive or steer your life. Remember you can be driven by your day or you can drive your day. The exercise below may take some time. I would suggest that you get away from your regular daily activities and work on this alone. This exercise is for you. If you follow God, get with God and ask for His wisdom. He will partner with you through this process.

Step 1: Write down all the things you do. All the hats you wear. All of your roles with responsibilities that you perform. If you are a working mother, you have more hats than a clown's dressing room. Write them all down. If you garden, you are your gardener. Write it all down. Don't leave anything out. Whether you are a working dad or unemployed at the time, or you are a stay at home mom or wife, you have plenty of roles. Whatever you are responsible to do, write it down.

Current roles/hats/responsibilities/tasks	Date hat last worn	Importance 1-10 (10 is most)

Step 2: Cross out anything on your list that does not coincide with your mission. Do this by putting one single line through them. You are not getting rid of them yet, just identifying them. This is going to be difficult because you may have been doing this for years. However, it needs to go if it doesn't get you to the place you want to be at the end of your life on earth. Let me give you an example.

If one of my roles is a softball player with the bros on Tuesday nights, but that doesn't fit my mission, then I need to quit the team. However, it may be a part of my mission to be a part of my community or to cultivate relationships or connect with people outside of church. If so, then I'll keep it. If it helps me fulfill my mission I'll keep doing it. We can't be afraid to quit things. Bob Goff in his book "Love Does" states that he quits something every Thursday. So quit if you need to.

After you do this, take a break, walk around, get a drink and then come back and look at the list with some freshness. Is there anything else that isn't on the highway to your mission?

Step 3: Looking at your list, circle the top three or four priorities and number their importance according to your mission. These top three or four things are special. This is where the 80/20 principle (aka the Pareto Principle) comes in which says that 80 percent of your goals can be accomplished by working on 20 percent of your tasks. Those top two to four things are where your time and energy need to go. According to the 80/20 principle, 80% of your energy should be spent in the top two or three priorities. This goes for your daily lists of to-dos as well. Look back at your top three roles and see how they will accomplish more than your numbers four through six. Do you have more top priorities than you can possibly give the proper amount of time and energy to? Some people have six top priorities! This means they don't have any real top priorities. They are still trying to squeeze everything into their life as a priority. This will lead to frustration and not being able to spend the proper time and energy on the top two or three priorities. If you have more than three or four top priorities, go back through the list and see if you can get rid of the lowest priority roles and responsibilities. I am not asking you to give up what you know you must do, I am urging you to reduce your list since you are not Michael Keaton in the movie Duplicity. He played a character that had clones. He got a lot done that way, but you are only one person. Make a list that reflects that fact.

Next, go through the list again and cross off the things that you really don't have to do. These are things that someone else could do. You may be able to pay someone to do that function or you could eliminate it altogether. For example, I could pay someone to do lawn care. Even if I like to do it, it gets in the way of other things that I have to do. Your mission is more important than liking an activity. If you like doing things like mowing the lawn, use it as personal time in your schedule. But for now, take things like that off your list. Also, you may consolidate a few things if need be, but they must be in the same category and be thought through concurrently.

Before you go on to Step 4 I want you to think about something. The most successful people in the world are learners. They spend time everyday learning. There are other habits like focused thinking and exercising that they make time for. I am not trying to create more roles, but surely one of your roles is taking care of yourself. My point is that you need to think about taking care of your personal growth and health as you plot out your schedule. The truly successful in life, not just in business, have contemplation or thoughtfulness time, creativity time, meditation or prayer time and other personal time. They do this so they can fulfill their mission, not for personal enjoyment, although it can be very enjoyable. You will want to remember these things again when it comes to plotting your week out. Did I just throw a monkey wrench in your priorities? You will thank me for the wrench later.

Step 4: Make a fresh list in order of priority of everything that is left—with the crossed-out roles (hats) at the bottom separated by a few blank lines above them. Your three to four main roles in order of importance should remain at the top of the list. This is the list that you will now use to create your Life Scheduling Template. This template will become your weekly and possibly a monthly living plan. You will create your daily schedules from this template with few exceptions. It is very important to whittle down your list. Again I stress the importance of the principle of time. As much as we wish there were, there are not more than 24 hours in a day and you have to sleep! You can't have 17 different things you do on your schedule because there will be no place to put them. Go back and try to get rid of as much as possible before you write this revised list.

Revised roles/hats/responsibilities/tasks	Date hat last worn	Importance 1-10 (10 is most)

Step 5: Put a line through the items on your revised list that you are willing to give up right now. Look over your nice, neat list that has the separation between the must wear hats and the things that someone else can do (even must do), and start crossing off some more items. Some may be troublesome to give up, or you may need to get someone to wear those hats. After you have simplified your life a little, or at least clarified your life, stand up and do a little dance!

Step 6: Categorize the things you must do according to your mission. Some of your responsibilities will now fall under categories that are clearly within your mission, or they will not. (If they do not, you will need to examine those roles and responsibilities closely and re-evaluate them.) Use your full 3-5 sentence mission statement for this exercise to assess which roles clearly fall within your mission. For example, I am a husband, a father and a healthly lifestyle influencer. These are all "missional roles" that come out of my overarching mission statement. Missional roles are the roles that fit directly into your clearly thought through mission statement. Missional roles are the top priorities in your life. You may have other roles from time to time that you must fufill, but if they don't fit into or get you to your stated destination, that role is a lower priority than the missional roles.

In the chart below you can see that writing this manual is a task that relates to my missional role of influencing people to live a remarkable life. Dating my wife is a part of my missional role to be a great husband. Being a good health coach (missonal role) fits into my overarching mission to influence people to live remarkably. Being a gardener or maintaining the lawn may be something that needs to be done, however, that doesn't mean I have to perform that role. I can pay a gardener to do that. It is so important to stick to the major things as you will discover when you complete this worksheet.

The purpose of categorizing your roles and responsibilities like this is it will be helpful for your Yearly Assignment coming up next. Remember to put any role that doesn't fit into your mission at the bottom of this worksheet. When do the steps end? When you have so fine-tuned your life that you live with maximal greatness in every area. I want you to live so great that even your rest is great! Someone will watch you taking a nap and say, "That guy/girl naps remarkably!"

Role	Missional role	Responsibilities/tasks
Author	*Influence people to live remarkable lives*	*Write TLP Life Manual*
Health Coach	*Influence people to live remarkable lives.*	*Regular workouts at the gym to help maintain great health as a great example.*
Husband	*Be a great husband*	*Regular dates with my wife*

You can probably guess what is next. Rewrite that list with the most important things—the top priorities, aka your missional roles in order of importance at the top of the list and the items that don't fit into your missional roles at the bottom of the list.

Role	Missional role	Responsibilities/tasks

Yearly Assignments

You may be tempted to skip this step, but I urge you to take the time to complete it. This step, like others, will take a considerable amount of time. Instead of a full cup of coffee or tea, you may need a carafe. (That's too much caffeine! Just drink water with a little lemon instead.) At this point, you should have a clearly defined overarching life mission, that include the different "missional roles" you operate in to fulfill that mission, along with an incredible reduction of the hats you wear in life. You have a purpose with roles that strategically align to your most important priorities in life.

Before you begin to plot your life on a calendar, it is wise to understand what that mission looks like this year. You will create goals to help you carry out your mission that may, and probably will, vary from year to year. Certainly, emphasis can change, and how you carry out your mission can change as well. So work through the following worksheet and list your goals for this year within each of the missional roles that you defined above from your overarching life mission.

I do want to say that sometimes we have certain responsibilities (that is a mission – think Navy Seal mission to rescue hostages) that don't last a lifetime. That really is a role that will fit into your life mission. Unlike being married or a parent, you could own a business and then sell it, or you could run a non-profit venture but eventually turn it over to a successor. Don't feel as if you can't have a role that is more temporary, and at this point it probably fits clearly within your mission.

Role	Goal	Tasks	Frequency/date
Health Coach	Gain new clients	Talk to five people	Per day

Now put _everything_ in priority. That means that your list is organized by your most important role and then it is sub-ordered by your most important task for that role.

Role	Goal	Task	Frequency/date
Health Coach	Gain new clients	Talk to five people	Per day

Life Scheduling Template

Your life plotted on a visual, functioning calendar is next. First, you will create a Life Scheduling Template. This template will give you an overarching baseline for your weekly and daily life. You may use a computer or write it out on the worksheet provided. (I recommend writing it out first). Start with the big things that just can't change first, such as sleep and work. Block those out. Planning your bedtime may seem like you are sending yourself to your room, but if you are a busy person, then you need to plan your sleep as well as everything else in your schedule. If you haven't worked on the *TLP Physical Manual* yet, apportioning four hours of sleep per night is not okay! Shoot for at least seven and a half which is five average sleep cycles. Absolutely no less than six hours no matter what!

After the non-negotiables, everything should be scheduled according to priority. Top priorities get the first shot at the time slots they need. There is an old video where Steven Covey is illustrating this with big rocks and little rocks. He has a woman dump a bunch of little rocks into a bucket and then asks her to put the big rocks into that same bucket. She fails because there is not enough room left in the bucket. That is our lives if we put all the small things we do first. When we try to fit in the big important things that absolutely are a part of our mission, we can't fit them into our day. There is no time left. Then he has her put the big rocks into the bucket first and then pour the little rocks in second. Almost all of the rocks now fit into the bucket. The point of the illustration is to put your big rocks, top priorities, mission critical tasks, into the bucket first. That is what I want you to do here.

After you fit (or haven't fit) everything in, go back and rework it. I like doing this in Excel or Word so I can color code things, which makes them stand out to me, but you can do it however you want. In fact, everyone is unique so you have to plan your schedule the way it will work for you, but don't use that as an excuse not to plan. Very few things are accomplished by accident (although I had seven children by accident, only one was planned). You can do this!

Note: I know that certain emergent or unforeseen things come up and will blow your day or week up. Travel, business meetings, graduations and the like happen. That is okay. This isn't the Law of Moses. What you are creating is a template to help you plan your life so the first things come first and you end up at your destination instead of the North Pole.

I understand in our electronic world that you may want to have this calendar on your phone, tablet, computer or all three as I do. However, I would encourage you to process this on paper to start. In fact, make a copy of the schedules first so you can erase, scribble and work through them more than once. There is something about seeing it all at once and writing down, erasing and figuring out what works best on paper. After you do that and get it all dialed in, then I encourage you to create a Word or Excel type calendar with colored blocks. I print mine out and put in on a board in my office to view all day every day.

Life Scheduling Template – Week 1

Time	Sun	Mon	Tue	Wed	Thur	Fri	Sat
6:00 am							
7:00 am							
8:00 am							
9:00 am							
10:00 am							
11:00 am							
12:00 pm							
1:00 pm							
2:00 pm							
3:00 pm							
4:00 pm							
5:00 pm							
6:00 pm							
7:00 pm							
8:00 pm							
9:00 pm							
10:00 pm							

Now go over your template one last time. Did you add in any free time or flex time? If not, go back and rework it. To have no flex time is to set yourself up for perfectionism, frustration or failure. You need some flex time. You can use it to produce or you can use it to relax. Speaking of relaxing...have you scheduled any purposeful relaxation time? Or recreation time? Or downtime? It is more important to your overall mission than you may think. Maybe you can use it to read a book or magazine or whatever. Just put it in your schedule. You will thank me later. One more thing. If you can't fit in all of your roles and priorities consider doing a two-week plan and you can alternate things from week to week. If you still can't fit it all in, then maybe you need to rethink your roles. You are only one person.

Okay, one more thing. If you have open gaps in your calendar, congratulations! Don't feel guilty. That's fantastic. Teach someone else how you did that. If you don't have gaps, fill out a new week 1 template on the following page as your final copy, until your roles change or you enter a new season, and you will make a new template for that season of life. I create a new template every year without looking at the old one. The big rocks are all in there like the previous year, however sometimes an emphasis may change. Also below you will find a second week option. Sometimes your life isn't the same every week. It changes because of your workflow or other reasons. Maybe you work three 12 hour days one week and four the next. Whatever the case, if you need a "week 2" Life Scheduling Template, use the Week 2 option. If not, leave it blank.

The Top 20%

Congratulations! You have just become one of the top 20% in the nation. You took the time, energy and effort to be more intentional and successful than ever. Now you get to walk it out. While your Life Scheduling Template that you just completed doesn't change from week to week (or every two weeks if you filled in the optional week two), your Weekly Appointment Calendar will. The wisdom here is that you will only schedule things on your Weekly Appointment Calendar that fit into your Life Scheduling Template.

We all know that emergencies happen, but you cannot afford to be ruled by the tyranny of the urgent. The great thing about having the template is that you had no emotionally charged issues or urgent deadlines when you birthed it. Now you can avoid the emotional decisions that are easy to make because of desires, demands, or because of the urgent or temporarily important. Make a promise to yourself that every week you will measure your Weekly Appointment Calendar against your Life Scheduling Template and make the necessary adjustments for them to align.

Life Scheduling Template – Week 1 (with flex-time)

Time	Sun	Mon	Tue	Wed	Thur	Fri	Sat
6:00 am							
7:00 am							
8:00 am							
9:00 am							
10:00 am							
11:00 am							
12:00 pm							
1:00 pm							
2:00 pm							
3:00 pm							
4:00 pm							
5:00 pm							
6:00 pm							
7:00 pm							
8:00 pm							
9:00 pm							
10:00 pm							

Life Scheduling Template – Week 2 (optional)

Time	Sun	Mon	Tue	Wed	Thur	Fri	Sat
6:00 am							
7:00 am							
8:00 am							
9:00 am							
10:00 am							
11:00 am							
12:00 pm							
1:00 pm							
2:00 pm							
3:00 pm							
4:00 pm							
5:00 pm							
6:00 pm							
7:00 pm							
8:00 pm							
9:00 pm							
10:00 pm							

Projects & Objectives

We have looked at your roles and responsibilities, your mission and your Life Scheduling Template and you are almost ready to begin filling in your Weekly Appointment Calendar. Most of us have projects that we must tend to. Whether you work for a company, or you are self-employed, or you are a full-time parent, your projects have to fit into your schedule. On a personal level, you may be working on a project at your house (e.g., building a Christmas present, or training for a 750-mile bike ride—I am presently planning for that) and you need it to work with your schedule. You may find that your current Life Scheduling Template doesn't allow for the necessary project time. You may see that you have too many projects to complete. Instead of stressing out about it, make a choice or make a change. You know what your "big rocks" are now. Your high priority items must remain high priority!

I remember sitting in a counseling session for our marriage, which evidently was all about me being stressed out. The counselor told me that I needed to think about leaving the pastorate. What? That was my life's work. I couldn't do that! He then gave me the other options. Change the way you live, change your vocation so you only have one job (I was bivocational—my income was also dependent upon work I did outside the church), or have a mental, emotional, or physical breakdown. What? He got my attention. I had to take another day off. I had to change. Sometimes things need to change to get to what you really want to do.

So the projects that you "have" to do..., do you have to? If so, put them in your schedule. Celebrate the fact that you will stay on your life's course if you complete the project.

Rather than trying to schedule an entire project that may take weeks, think of it in terms of smaller objectives. If you want to put in a new countertop and cupboards, break it down into bite-size daily and or week objectives. Once you have your objectives for the day or week, then you can schedule them. For example, instead of having the main objective of getting a new counter and new cupboards installed next week, break it down into smaller steps such as contacting a contractor, picking out the style of cupboards, etc. Break it down into as many steps as you can so you can more accurately predict the actual time that those objectives will take.

There are many great project organizers out there, you can choose one of them or you can use the worksheet below. Remember that your objective is to accurately predict how long the project will take and insert that into your Daily & Weekly Appointment Calendar so long as it aligns with your Life Scheduling Template. You are not superperson so, be realistic with your estimates and give plenty of time for unexpected and uncontrollable circumstances.

Main Objective Worksheet

Instructions:

1. Decide on the main objective of your larger project goal.

2. List all of the major objectives required to obtain your main objective.

3. Next, assign an order to the major objectives if they are out of order.

4. List the minor objectives that it will take to complete the major objectives—be thorough.

5. Use the worksheet to plot these tasks according to your Life Scheduling Template on your Daily & Weekly Appointment Schedules. You may go as far in advance as you want, however, be flexible for setbacks, especially when you are waiting on other people before you can continue.

Example:

Project: Get new countertops and cupboards for the kitchen

Main Objective: Hire a contractor

Priority	Major Objective	Minor Objectives
1	*Get references*	*Talk to neighbors*
		Check local ads, online
		Check reviews online
2	*Get estimates*	*Gather contact info of potential companies*
		Make phone calls to schedule an initial appointment
3	*Hire the contractor*	*Assess the estimates*
		Call chosen contractor to set up the project start day

Main Objective Worksheet

Project: _____

Main Objective: _____

_____

_____

Priority	Major Objective	Minor Objectives

Planning Your Week

You have your Life Scheduling Template in front of you and now you get to fill in your Weekly Appointment Calendar. This is *not* a template, this is everything that you *will do* the week of September 2, etc. When things come up that don't have a slot, you are going to have to make a choice and sometimes that choice is going to be, "I'm sorry, I won't be able to do that." Say that out loud. Okay, repeat it one more time. Now say it to yourself in the mirror. For most of us that is so hard to say. We don't want to disappoint anyone or make them upset with us. *Someone* may get upset, but you get to choose who.

When I have a date night scheduled with my honey of 34 years and someone calls me and needs me to do some marriage counseling because they are in crisis, I get to choose who gets upset. I can tell you that it won't be my wife, nor myself, for doing the counseling. I have given up my date night before for a crisis. A family in our church got bad news about their daughter who had been fighting cancer for over a year. It had spread. They were in pieces. My wife and I both wanted to go sit with them instead of having a date. We did, and we weren't upset. My point is, I get to choose. My date night is on my calendar and therefore you better have some good hockey tickets if you want to cut in on that time. (And you better have four seats so I can bring my wife.)

You have to weed out and delegate those things that don't belong on your weekly or daily schedule. Have a place to write those things down, because I know these items still need to be accomplished, it's just that you aren't going to do them. Some would say it takes too long if someone else does it, and I can do it better and faster anyway. I know. I agree. Delegate it or dump it. It can't fit on your very important schedule.

Again, I encourage you to fill out the calendars with a pencil. I do want you to keep a calendar on all of your devices and put detailed information in the note section of every appointment for easy reference, however, work it out with a pencil on the sheets provided first, and then transfer it to the electronic format.

Weekly Appointment Calendar – Week 1:

Time	Sun	Mon	Tue	Wed	Thur	Fri	Sat
6:00 am							
7:00 am							
8:00 am							
9:00 am							
10:00 am							
11:00 am							
12:00 pm							
1:00 pm							
2:00 pm							
3:00 pm							
4:00 pm							
5:00 pm							
6:00 pm							
7:00 pm							
8:00 pm							
9:00 pm							
10:00 pm							

Week 1 Assessment

You are through your first week. Great job! Now, take a look back at the week. Did you keep all of your calendared items on point? Go through and notate what really happened if what your calendar says didn't come to pass.

Now compare all the corrections you noted on your Weekly Appointment Calendar to your Life Scheduling Template. Put them side by side.

What percentage of your Weekly Appointment Calendar aligns with your Life Scheduling Template? _____

Of your three to four highest priority roles, what percentage of your actual Weekly Appointment Calendar was spent on those roles? _____

What was most of your time spent doing? _____

Does that accurately reflect your Life Scheduling Template? _____

What adjustments could you make to next week to ensure that more of your Weekly Appointment Calendar stays focused on your most important roles?

_____

_____

_____

_____

_____

Week 2 is coming up, make sure your Weekly Appointment Calendar is filled in before the week starts.

Weekly Appointment Calendar – Week 2:

Time	Sun	Mon	Tue	Wed	Thur	Fri	Sat
6:00 am							
7:00 am							
8:00 am							
9:00 am							
10:00 am							
11:00 am							
12:00 pm							
1:00 pm							
2:00 pm							
3:00 pm							
4:00 pm							
5:00 pm							
6:00 pm							
7:00 pm							
8:00 pm							
9:00 pm							
10:00 pm							

Week 2 Assessment

Take a look back at the week. Did you keep all of your calendared items on point? Go through and notate what really happened if what your calendar isn't 100% accurate.

Now compare all the corrections you noted on your Weekly Appointment Calendar to your Life Scheduling Template. Put them side by side.

What percentage of your Weekly Appointment Calendar aligns with your Life Scheduling Template? _____

Of your three to four highest priority roles, what percentage of your actual Weekly Appointment Calendar was spent on those roles? _____

What was most of your time spent doing? _____

Does that accurately reflect your Life Scheduling Template? _____

What adjustments could you make to next week to ensure that more of your Weekly Appointment Calendar stays focused on your most important roles?

_____

_____

_____

_____

_____

Week 3 is coming up, make sure your Weekly Appointment Calendar is filled in before the week starts.

Weekly Appointment Calendar – Week 3:

Time	Sun	Mon	Tue	Wed	Thur	Fri	Sat
6:00 am							
7:00 am							
8:00 am							
9:00 am							
10:00 am							
11:00 am							
12:00 pm							
1:00 pm							
2:00 pm							
3:00 pm							
4:00 pm							
5:00 pm							
6:00 pm							
7:00 pm							
8:00 pm							
9:00 pm							
10:00 pm							

Week 3 Assessment

Take a look back at your week. Did you keep all of your calendared items on point? Go through and notate what really happened if what your calendar says isn't accurate.

Now compare all the corrections you noted on your Weekly Appointment Calendar to your Life Scheduling Template. Put them side by side.

What percentage of your Weekly Appointment Calendar aligns with your Life Scheduling Template? _____

Of your three to four highest priority roles, what percentage of your actual Weekly Appointment Calendar was spent on those roles? _____

Using colored highlighters, color code your Life Scheduling Template. Use a different color for each different role. Now go to your Weekly Appointment Calendar and color your time blocks in with the coordinating color of the role that you operated within.

What was most of your time spent doing? _____

Does that accurately reflect your Life Scheduling Template? _____

What adjustments could you make to next week to ensure that more of your Weekly Appointment Calendar stays focused on your most important roles?

_____

_____

_____

_____

_____

Week 4 is coming up, make sure your Weekly Appointment Calendar is filled in before the week starts. Before you write anything down, color coordinate it with your Life Scheduling Template. Hopefully, you have built in some blank spaces. Leave those white. Now fill in the actual scheduled appointments and tasks for the week and stay within the colors of your Life Scheduling Template unless an urgent and important matter arises.

Weekly Appointment Calendar – Week 4:

Time	Sun	Mon	Tue	Wed	Thur	Fri	Sat
6:00 am							
7:00 am							
8:00 am							
9:00 am							
10:00 am							
11:00 am							
12:00 pm							
1:00 pm							
2:00 pm							
3:00 pm							
4:00 pm							
5:00 pm							
6:00 pm							
7:00 pm							
8:00 pm							
9:00 pm							
10:00 pm							

Week 4 Assessment

How did you do on week four? Grade yourself with an A to F system: _____

Are you happy with that grade? _____

Is there anything that you can do moving forward to stay aligned with your mission better? (Think dump and delegate, or think about making a schedule that a human can perform). If there are revisions to your Life Scheduling Template, make them now. Just remember to stay on *mission*!

_____

_____

_____

_____

_____

_____

_____

_____

_____

_____

_____

_____

_____

_____

Organization

I have something that needs to go on your calendar somewhere. Organizing your desk or workspace. Decluttering your life is part of what this exercise does. I know, I know, some people work better with a messy desk. Your desk should be indicative of your focus, life and schedule. Singular. Purposeful. Orderly. Start with the top of your desks and then organize your drawers. Get rid of the stuff you don't need. Give the things that you delegated to the person you passed the related task to. The things you need to keep can go into a file. Neatly. Then you can pull it out when you work on that project.

I know this is going to be a stretch, but organize your office or workspace area. When your area has 20 different things all over the place, it tends to pull you in too many different directions and you lose focus. I am not talking about 20 different books, I am talking about files on top of files, papers here and there, stacks of stuff...trash. If you are a messy person, welcome to having a workplace that is organized and looks like your life. Make sure this is on your Life Scheduling Template, if necessary, so it remains tidy.

To-dos

Everyone needs a to-do list. Besides being a way to ensure the important tasks get done, it is a way to mentally dump all those things you are trying to remember to do. This is a great stress reducer. Please reread the last two sentences. A to-do list is a stress reducer! That is reason enough to have one. The other reason is that it is great to have a visible list of what and when you need to accomplish things.

At the beginning of every week, go through your to-do list and (guess what I am going to say) dump or delegate what you can. (Repetitive, I know. But you need to get the principle). It will become fun to cross off the things you thought you *needed to do*, but really didn't need to do. Prioritize the rest of the items based on importance, dependence and urgency. When one task needs to get done to get to other tasks (e.g., fill the car with gas before you leave for a road trip), that task goes to the front of the line. Get the big ones out of the way first. The most successful people tackle the hard things that they don't necessarily like first, as long as it lands high on your to-do list scale. You get to decide which of those are based on mission, urgency, importance and dependency. It will be helpful to prioritize your to-do list before adding them to your schedule. I know that can be tough at times so I have included a Task Priority Matrix later in this manual.

After prioritizing your to-do items, you are ready to put them in your schedule. Caution! You may run out of time. You may have too many to-do items and they won't all fit in your calendar. If it won't fit in your calendar, it won't fit in your life. Don't load your calendar with things you don't have the time to accomplish. Does that make sense? We take on too many tasks that will take us years to get to and then continue to take on tasks. That has got to stop! It stresses us all out. Practice saying no again if you need to. Do it, delegate it or dump it! You get to choose what gets done and what doesn't. You can put them off until next week or next month or...you could delegate or dump them.

On the following worksheet, list your to-do items and if there is a deadline. If you are clear on the urgency, importance, dependency and what it means in your life, then assign a priority to it. In the delegate column, put the person's name who this task will be delegated to if you know who you will ask. Otherwise, dump it and feel good about that.

There are many to-do lists out there for electronic devices. Evernote is a popular one as is To-doist. Asana and others are more like project managers. You may like that approach better. Choose one that easily sync's with all of your devices and is easy to use. The one thing that most of them lack is priority. You will have to figure out how to prioritize them based on your criteria with the wisdom of Solomon.

To-Do List

Item	Due	Priority	Delegate	Dump

To-Do List

Item	Due	Priority	Delegate	Dump

To-Do List

Item	Due	Priority	Delegate	Dump

To-Do List

Item	Due	Priority	Delegate	Dump

Task Matrix

This is a tool that takes the *big* decision and makes it into many small decisions. Sometimes this is really helpful especially when you are emotionally charged or have a predisposition to obsess over decisions. You can use this to understand the true priority that a given task should have.

Example Task Matrix:

Task	Value 0-8	Value 0-8	No=5 Yes=0	No=0 Yes=3	No=0 Yes=3	Value 0-5	Value 0-10	Total
	Deadline approaching	Importance	Can I delegate it?	Are others dependent on it?	Are other tasks dependent on it?	Will it relieve stress?	Will it help me fulfill my mission?	
Create TLP Life Manual	3	8	5	0	4	4	10	34
Get TLP DBA	5	5	0	0	4	2	2	18
Update TLP website	8	8	0	0	0	3	3	22

Task Matrix Worksheet

Task	Value 0-8	Value 0-8	No=5 Yes=0	No=0 Yes=3	No=0 Yes=3	Value 0-5	Value 0-10	Total
	Deadline approaching	Importance	Can I delegate it?	Are others dependent on it?	Are other tasks dependent on it?	Will it relieve stress?	Will it help me fulfill my mission?	

Task Matrix Worksheet

Task	Value 0-8	Value 0-8	No=5 Yes=0	No=0 Yes=3	No=0 Yes=3	Value 0-5	Value 0-10	Total
	Deadline approaching	Importance	Can I delegate it?	Are others dependent on it?	Are other tasks dependent on it?	Will it relieve stress?	Will it help me fulfill my mission?	

Progress Assessment

Before we get to the next two sections, how has it been going? Have you grown? Have you stepped up a level or two or more? I would wager that you have. You are that kind of person. Here are a couple of questions that may help you see that things are changing.

My life and my weekly/daily schedules are more intentional and planned: Yes   or   No

How are you living differently day to day than you were before you began this manual?

_____

_____

_____

Did you get a good handle on your life mission(s)?	0	1	2	3	4	5
Are you dumping and delegating more?	0	1	2	3	4	5
Are you finding that your schedule has come under more control rather than controlling you?	0	1	2	3	4	5
Has there been a time when you have said no to something because it didn't fit in your schedule?	0	1	2	3	4	5
Do you know when your next vacation is?	0	1	2	3	4	5
Did you schedule (and then keep) your rest and fun time better than before you started?	0	1	2	3	4	5

Goals

Thinking about the four quadrants, what percentage of time do you want to spend in each quadrant?

Quadrant 1: _____

Quadrant 2: _____

Quadrant 3: _____

Quadrant 4: _____

At the end of the week when you look back at your Weekly Appointment Calendar, what percentage of staying true to your calendar would you consider success?

_____

_____

_____

If there was an overall goal for this area of your life—life planning—what would it be?

_____

_____

_____

Create 3-5 goals to be attained this year that pertain to your mission and to your specific roles. These goals should pertain to your mission and to your specific roles. Make sure each goal meets the SMART acronym model (Specific, Measurable, Achievable, Relevant, Time Sensitive). I've included a brief reminder of this for you to follow here.

Specific – Write very specific goals that anyone would be able to understand.
Measurable – Measure your goals with some kind of metric. If it can't be measured, then it isn't a goal.
Achievable – The goal has to reside on planet earth. Keep your goals to things that can actually happen.
Relevant – The goals have to be relevant to your mission.
Time Sensitive – There has to be a specific date or hour when these goals will be achieved.

Goal Worksheet

Articulate a specific goal:

_____

_____

_____

_____

_____

How will you measure it?

_____

_____

_____

List four stages of progress on the way to the goal:

1. _____

2. _____

3. _____

4. _____

Is your goal actually doable?

_____

_____

_____

Is it relevant to your life mission and planning?

_____

_____

_____

_____

_____

_____

When will it be accomplished? _____

Goal Worksheet

Articulate a specific goal:

_____

_____

_____

_____

_____

How will you measure it?

_____

_____

_____

List four stages of progress on the way to the goal:

1. _____

2. _____

3. _____

4. _____

Is your goal actually doable?

_____

_____

_____

Is it relevant to your life mission and planning?

_____

_____

_____

_____

_____

_____

When will it be accomplished? _____

Goal Worksheet

Articulate a specific goal:

_____

_____

_____

_____

_____

How will you measure it?

_____

_____

_____

List four stages of progress on the way to the goal:

1. _____

2. _____

3. _____

4. _____

Is your goal actually doable?

_____

_____

_____

Is it relevant to your life mission and planning?

_____

_____

_____

_____

_____

_____

When will it be accomplished? _____

Goal Worksheet

Articulate a specific goal:

_____

_____

_____

_____

_____

How will you measure it?

_____

_____

_____

List four stages of progress on the way to the goal:

1. _____

2. _____

3. _____

4. _____

Is your goal actually doable?

_____

_____

_____

Is it relevant to your life mission and planning?

_____

_____

_____

_____

_____

_____

When will it be accomplished? _____

Goal Worksheet

Articulate a specific goal:

_____

_____

_____

_____

_____

How will you measure it?

_____

_____

_____

List four stages of progress on the way to the goal:

1. _____

2. _____

3. _____

4. _____

Is your goal actually doable?

_____

_____

_____

Is it relevant to your life mission and planning?

_____

_____

_____

_____

_____

_____

When will it be accomplished? _____

Goal Worksheet

Articulate a specific goal:

_____

_____

_____

_____

_____

How will you measure it?

_____

_____

_____

List four stages of progress on the way to the goal:

1. _____

2. _____

3. _____

4. _____

Is your goal actually doable?

_____

_____

_____

Is it relevant to your life mission and planning?

_____

_____

_____

_____

_____

_____

When will it be accomplished? _____

Gratefulness

There is one last thing I want to encourage you to include in your daily life. I promise you it will produce big dividends. Gratefulness. Did you know your brain has a bent towards gratitude? It is true! You are designed for it and now research shows that everything is better in your brain and body if you are grateful. The opposite of gratefulness is criticism. An attitude of criticism is a negative view of the events of the day or week that did not go perfectly or to plan. That is not needed and is not helpful in the least. What is helpful is choosing gratitude for your wins. That creates homeostasis in your brain and allows you to think better. That is helpful for production and for life! So let's do it! At the end of every day and every week write down what you are grateful for. Do not make it something like, I am thankful that I didn't totally collapse. Find a win and celebrate it. Let the accomplishment propel you to more of it!

When you fill out the next four pages with grateful things, avoid repetitious items except when you are being very purposeful in repeating something that you are grateful for. I am asking you to think deeply rather than write down the first few things that come into your head every day. You may copy the following page and use it as much as you would like.

Gratefulness Journal – Week 1

Date:_____   Today I am thankful for_____

_____

_____

Date:_____   Today I am thankful for_____

_____

_____

Date:_____   Today I am thankful for_____

_____

_____

Date:_____   Today I am thankful for_____

_____

_____

Date:_____   Today I am thankful for_____

_____

_____

Date:_____   Today I am thankful for_____

_____

_____

Date:_____   Today I am thankful for_____

_____

_____

This week I am thankful for_____

_____

_____

_____

_____

_____

_____

_____

Gratefulness Journal – Week 2

Date:_____ Today I am thankful for_____

_____

_____

Date:_____ Today I am thankful for_____

_____

_____

Date:_____ Today I am thankful for_____

_____

_____

Date:_____ Today I am thankful for_____

_____

_____

Date:_____ Today I am thankful for_____

_____

_____

Date:_____ Today I am thankful for_____

_____

_____

Date:_____ Today I am thankful for_____

_____

This week I am thankful for_____

_____

_____

_____

_____

_____

_____

Gratefulness Journal – Week 3

Date:_____ Today I am thankful for_____

_____

_____

Date:_____ Today I am thankful for_____

_____

_____

Date:_____ Today I am thankful for_____

_____

_____

Date:_____ Today I am thankful for_____

_____

_____

Date:_____ Today I am thankful for_____

_____

_____

Date:_____ Today I am thankful for_____

_____

_____

Date:_____ Today I am thankful for_____

_____

_____

This week I am thankful for_____

_____

_____

_____

_____

_____

_____

_____

Gratefulness Journal – Week 4

Date:_____ Today I am thankful for_____

_____

_____

Date:_____ Today I am thankful for_____

_____

_____

Date:_____ Today I am thankful for_____

_____

_____

Date:_____ Today I am thankful for_____

_____

_____

Date:_____ Today I am thankful for_____

_____

_____

Date:_____ Today I am thankful for_____

_____

_____

Date:_____ Today I am thankful for_____

_____

_____

This week I am thankful for_____

_____

_____

_____

_____

_____

_____

Reflection

Sometimes we grow and never acknowledge that growth. We have this starting place, let's call it D. We purposefully live life and spend time growing so we raise up to level M. I think it is wise to acknowledge it and thank God for the growth. Some people are well below the level they could be operating at in life. You are making progress. Take the time to reflect on your time spent working through this manual, evaluating your life and planning it out.

What did you learn? _____

_____

_____

_____

_____

_____

_____

_____

_____

_____

_____

_____

_____

_____

_____

_____

_____

_____

_____

_____

_____

_____

_____

How did you grow? _____

_____

_____

_____

_____

_____

_____

_____

_____

_____

_____

_____

_____

_____

_____

_____

_____

_____

_____

_____

_____

_____

_____

_____

_____

What surprised you?

_____

_____

_____

_____

_____

_____

_____

_____

_____

_____

_____

_____

_____

_____

_____

_____

_____

_____

_____

_____

_____

_____

_____

_____

_____

What delighted you? _____

_____

_____

_____

_____

_____

_____

_____

_____

_____

_____

_____

_____

_____

_____

_____

_____

_____

_____

_____

_____

_____

_____

_____

_____

_____

_____

_____

What are you looking forward to next? _____

_____
_____
_____
_____
_____
_____
_____
_____
_____
_____
_____
_____
_____
_____
_____
_____
_____
_____
_____
_____
_____
_____
_____
_____
_____
_____
_____

Congratulations! You are done, until tomorrow, next week, or next year! Obviously, your weekly schedule needs daily or weekly attention. I suggest filling out your schedule for next week and your to-do list before the end of the current week. You will be able to prioritize things better. Also, I encourage you to get away for at least a day, if not two, when it comes time to think about the next year's Life Scheduling Template. Your priorities may change or you may discover a need that you hadn't seen before. How you are going to accomplish things certainly will change, and those changes need to be accounted and planned for. Go camping, book a local hotel, just get away so you can think clearly without distraction from your current schedule.

There are other things that I could have included to help you with your life planning, however, this is your beginning, or part of your journey. You will discover more tools as you go. When you find one you like, utilize it! You've done well. Keep up the good work! Greatness awaits.

Live Remarkably!

Total Life Pursuit Workshops

Terry Miller is available for booking for your group, company or church. Terry currently hosts three types of workshops and various talks about health, wellness and relationships as well as Health Coaching. Reach out for more information on any of the following workshops and be sure to follow TLP for more insights and education. If there is another topic you would like to hear from Terry, please send him and the TLP team your suggestion. Terry is passionate to bring the wealth of the TLP lifestyle to all who want it. Connect with him today!

Health Made Simple Workshop
This workshop can be done in a standalone format of three to six hours, or may be offered as a culture shift event – a week-long event with classes, private trainings, staff courses and the workshop. This workshop will walk your group, company or church through Terry's Four Pillars of Health in an informative, engaging and practical way.

Life Planning Workshop
This workshop takes the principles in the *TLP Starting Line* manual, along with many examples and inspirational stories, and walks you through the steps of understanding your purpose and how to plan in order to effectively live out your calling in life.

Romance Saved My Marriage Workshop
This workshop helps married couples remember the good reasons they chose to get married and rekindle or fan the flame of passion in their marriage.

Health Talks
This 45-minute presentation focuses on empowering people to make the decisions that are needed to create a lifestyle of greater health and fitness.

Life Talks
Terry speaks on a wide variety of topics to empower and inspire people to live a remarkable life.

Health Coaching vs. Personal Training
Personal training is specific to fitness and mobility goals. There is no doubt that you will become healthier through becoming more fit, but personal training emphasizes foundational strength and stability, movement, mobility, strength training and endurance training. Health coaching utilizes all of the above, but adds into it the concept of overall health and wellness and lifestyle change. Health coaching takes into account all of your physical history and Terry can work with your physicians to bring about a cohesive approach to your health and wellness. Terry brings his four pillars of health to his coaching to bring about remarkable health in your life.

Contact us: *totallifepursuit@gmail.com*

Check out our blog: *totallifepursuit.org/blog*

 @totallifepursuit

 Total Life Pursuit

Made in United States
Cleveland, OH
06 June 2025